97 Meal and Juice Recipes to Increase Your Energy and Feel Great:

Eliminate Fatigue and Low Energy during the Day

By

Joe Correa CSN

COPYRIGHT

ACKNOWLEDGEMENTS

This book is dedicated to my friends and family that have had mild or serious illnesses so that you may find a solution and make the necessary changes in your life.

97 Meal and Juice Recipes to Increase Your Energy and Feel Great:

Eliminate Fatigue and Low Energy during the Day

By

Joe Correa CSN

CONTENTS

ABOUT THE AUTHOR

After years of Research, I honestly believe in the positive effects that proper nutrition can have over the body and mind. My knowledge and experience has helped me live healthier throughout the years and which I have shared with family and friends. The more you know about eating and drinking healthier, the sooner you will want to change your life and eating habits.

Nutrition is a key part in the process of being healthy and living longer so get started today. The first step is the most important and the most significant.

INTRODUCTION

97 Meal and Juice Recipes to Increase Your Energy and Feel Great: Eliminate Fatigue and Low Energy during the Day

By Joe Correa CSN

Food is life, our main source of energy, and our driving force. You don't have to be an expert to understand that we need to eat in order to survive. Nutrients we consume through food supply our body with energy and give us the strength to perform everyday tasks.

However, unhealthy eating habits, poor diet, and the lack of nutrients will cause a lack of energy and fatigue. These conditions not only affect our physical well-being, but they are also related to so many different emotional conditions which lead to a complete immune system break down. Consequently, we are opening the door to so many acute and chronic diseases, medical conditions, and infections. Without any doubt, I can say that the way we eat affects our entire life.

Based on my personal experience and extensive research, I created a collection of recipes that will be perfect protein boosters for overall physical energy, but also high in vitamins and minerals for a nutritionally stocked day which will help you to feel full of energy even with a busy schedule.

The recipes you will find in this book are based on fresh fruits and vegetables, lean meats, legumes, nuts, and seeds. At the same time, I wanted to keep the recipes simple, without any complicated procedures.

Remember that your overall health is a direct reflection of the foods you eat. It defines us in all possible ways and the energy that we get from it guides us towards better health, happiness, and success. A combination of a proper diet, regular physical activity, avoiding alcohol and cigarettes are the only true ways to solving the unwanted side effects of poor dietary habits like the overall lack of energy and fatigue.

Prepare these recipes every day and enjoy every bite.

97 MEAL AND JUICE RECIPES TO INCREASE YOUR ENERGY AND FEEL GREAT: ELIMINATE FATIGUE AND LOW ENERGY DURING THE DAY

MEALS

1.   Bean Veal Stew

Ingredients:

1 lb of lean veal, cut into bite-sized pieces

1 lb of kidney beans

1 cup of tomatoes, finely chopped

1 large potato, peeled and cubed

1 large yellow bell pepper, chopped

1 small onion, finely chopped

2 garlic cloves, crushed

3 tbsp of olive oil

1 tsp of dried thyme, ground

4 cups of chicken broth

½ tsp of pink Himalayan salt

½ tsp of black pepper, ground

Preparation:

Wash the meat under cold running water and pat dry with a kitchen paper. Cut into bite-sized pieces and set aside.

Preheat the oil in a large heavy-bottomed pot over a medium-high temperature. Add garlic and onion and cook for 3 minutes, or until slightly translucent. Add meat and cook for 10 minutes, or until golden browned. Reduce the heat to low and pour 1 cup of broth. Stir occasionally.

Wash and prepare the vegetables. Add potato, tomatoes, and bell pepper. Cook for 10 minutes and then season with thyme, salt, and pepper. Add remaining broth and stir well. Cook for 30 minutes, or until set.

Remove from the heat and serve warm.

Nutrition information per serving: Kcal: 322, Protein: 24.4g, Carbs: 37.2g, Fats: 8.8g

2.   Asparagus with Hollandaise Sauce

Ingredients:

2 lbs of wild asparagus, trimmed and chopped

2 large onion, sliced

2 large egg yolks, beaten

2 tbsp of butter, melted

4 garlic cloves, crushed

3 tbsp of olive oil

2 tbsp of lemon juice, freshly squeezed

½ tsp of salt

¼ tsp of black pepper

Preparation:

Wash the asparagus under cold running water and trim off the woody ends. Cut into bite-sized pieces and set aside.

In a medium-sized bowl, combine melted butter, egg yolks, lemon juice, salt, and pepper. Stir well to blend and set aside.

Preheat the oil in a large saucepan over a medium-high temperature. Add onions and garlic and cook for 3-4 minutes, or until translucent. Add asparagus and stir all well to combine. Add about 4 tablespoons of water and cook for 6-8 minutes, or until asparagus nicely soften. Remove from the heat and transfer to serving plates. Reserve the pan.

Pour the sauce mixture into a pan and cook for 2 minutes on low temperature, stirring constantly.

Drizzle the asparagus with sauce and enjoy!

Nutrition information per serving: Kcal: 143, Protein: 4.3g, Carbs: 9.9g, Fats: 10.8g

3.   Nut Banana Smoothie

Ingredients:

1 tbsp of almonds

1 tbsp of walnuts

1 tbsp of cashews

1 large egg yolk

1 large banana, chopped

1 cup almond yogurt

1 tsp of vanilla extract

1 tbsp of honey

Preparation:

Combine all ingredients in a food processor and blend until nicely smooth. Transfer to a serving glass and refrigerate for 20 minutes before serving.

Enjoy!

Nutrition information per serving: Kcal: 214, Protein: 11.2g, Carbs: 33.8g, Fats: 9.7g

4.   Avocado Pineapple Salad

Ingredients:

1 cup of avocado chunks

1 cup of pineapple chunks

1 cup of watermelon

1 cup of sour cream

1 cup of spinach, finely chopped

1 tbsp of honey

1 tsp of vanilla extract

1 tbsp of flaxseeds

Preparation:

In a medium bowl, combine sour cream, honey, vanilla extract, and flaxseeds. Stir well to combine and set aside.

Wash and prepare the vegetables.

Peel the avocado and pineapple and cut in half. Remove the pit from the avocado and cut into small chunks along with pineapple. Place in a large salad bowl and set aside.

Cut one large watermelon wedge and peel it. Cut into bite-sized pieces and discard the seeds. Add it to the bowl with other fruits and set aside.

Wash the spinach thoroughly under cold running water and roughly chop it. Add it to the bowl with other fruits.

Now, pour the sour cream mixture over the fruits and veggies and toss well to coat all the ingredients.

Refrigerate for 15 minutes before serving.

Nutrition information per serving: Kcal: 346, Protein: 4.7g, Carbs: 25.5g, Fats: 26.5g

5.   Juicy Lamb Chops

Ingredients:

1 lb of lamb chops

2 medium-sized red bell peppers, chopped

1 small onion, sliced

1 cup of sweet potatoes, cubed

4 garlic cloves, finely chopped

1 tsp of salt

1 tsp of dried thyme, ground

1 tsp of cayenne pepper, ground

3 cups of bone broth

2 tbsp of oil

1 tbsp of butter, melted

Preparation:

Preheat the oven to 325°F.

Wash the meat under cold running water and pat dry with a kitchen paper. Rub the meat with some salt and set aside.

Preheat the oil in a large nonstick skillet over a medium-high temperature. Add meat chops and cook for 5 minutes on each side, or until golden brown. Remove from the heat and set aside.

Melt the butter in a microwave and brush a large baking sheet. Place the meat in the middle and coat with vegetables. Pour the vegetable broth and season with thyme, cayenne pepper, garlic, salt, and pepper.

Place it in the oven and cook for 1 hour, or until vegetables tender. Remove from the oven and serve warm.

Nutrition information per serving: Kcal: 268, Protein: 24.8g, Carbs: 12.5g, Fats: 12.9g

6. Spinach Onion Soup

Ingredients:

1 lb of spinach, finely chopped

4 garlic cloves, crushed

3 cups of vegetable broth

1 small onion, chopped

1 cup of sour cream

2 tbsp of butter

½ tsp of salt

¼ tsp of black pepper, ground

Preparation:

Wash the spinach thoroughly under cold running water. Chop it into small pieces and set aside.

Melt the butter in a heavy-bottomed pot over a medium-high temperature. Add onion and garlic and stir-fry until translucent. Pour in the vegetable broth and add spinach. Season with salt and pepper to taste, and bring it to a boil. Reduce the heat to low and cook for 15 more minutes.

Stir in the sour cream and cook until heated thoroughly. Remove from the heat and serve warm.

Nutrition information per serving: Kcal: 160, Protein: 6.1g, Carbs: 6.6g, Fats: 12.9g

7. Turkey-Saffron Pate

Ingredients:

2 lbs of turkey breasts, skinless and boneless

1 cup of chicken broth

¼ tsp of saffron

1 tsp of salt

1 tbsp of Dijon mustard

2 tbsp of olive oil

Preparation:

Wash the breasts under cold running water and pat dry with a kitchen paper. Cut into bite-sized pieces and set aside.

Preheat the oil in a large nonstick skillet over a medium-high temperature. Add meat and sprinkle with some salt. Cook for 5 minutes, stirring occasionally.

Add chicken broth and stir in the mustard and saffron. Bring it to a boil and then reduce the heat to low. Cook for 3 minutes and remove from the heat. Set aside to cool completely.

Transfer all to a food processor and blend until well combined and pureed. Serve with whole wheat bread slices.

Nutrition information per serving: Kcal: 268, Protein: 24.8g, Carbs: 12.5g, Fats: 12.9g

8.   Quinoa with Veggies

Ingredients:

2 cups of quinoa, pre-cooked

1 large red bell pepper, chopped

2 large carrots, sliced

2 tbsp of fresh parsley, finely chopped

1 tsp of salt

1 cup of sweet potatoes, cubed

1 large tomato, diced

3 tbsp of olive oil

1 tsp of cayenne pepper, ground

1 cup of chicken broth

Preparation:

Place the quinoa in a deep pot and add 4 cups of water. Bring it to a boil and then reduce the heat to low. Cook for 15 minutes, stirring occasionally. Remove from the heat and set aside.

Preheat the oil in a large nonstick skillet over a medium-high temperature. Add carrots and potatoes and sprinkle with a pinch of salt. Cook for 5 minutes and then add chicken broth. Bring it to a boil and stir in the tomato. Cook for 1 minute and then add quinoa. Sprinkle with parsley, cayenne pepper and salt. Stir well and cook for 5 more minutes. If you like it juicier, add ½ cup of broth and cook for 5 minutes longer.

Remove from the heat and serve warm.

Enjoy!

Nutrition information per serving: Kcal: 393, Protein: 11.9g, Carbs: 58.5g, Fats: 13g

9. Creamy Salmon Omelet

Ingredients:

1 lb of salmon fillets, cut into bite-sized pieces

4 large eggs, beaten

1 large onion, chopped

2 tbsp of olive oil

1 tsp of fresh rosemary, finely chopped

½ cup of Greek yogurt

1 garlic clove, crushed

1 tsp of apple cider vinegar

2 tbsp of fresh parsley finely chopped

1 tsp of sea salt

Preparation:

Wash the fillets under cold running water and pat dry with a kitchen paper. Cut into bite-sized pieces. Sprinkle with salt and set aside.

In a medium bowl, combine yogurt, garlic, vinegar, and parsley. Stir well to blend and set aside.

Preheat the oil in a large frying pan over a medium-high temperature. Add onions and stir-fry for about 3-4 minutes, or until translucent. Add meat and cook for 3 minutes, stirring occasionally. Now, pour beaten eggs and cook for 4 minutes or until eggs are set. Remove from the heat.

Spoon the sour cream mixture onto one half of the omelet and fold. Serve immediately.

Nutrition information per serving: Kcal: 323, Protein: 31.9g, Carbs: 5.7g, Fats: 19.7g

10.   Basmati Chicken

Ingredients:

1 lb of chicken fillets, cut into bite-sized pieces

1 cup of basmati rice, pre-cooked

1 large red bell pepper, chopped

1 tsp of turmeric, ground

1 tsp of salt

1 tbsp of fresh parsley, finely chopped

¼ tsp of black pepper, ground

1 ½ cup of chicken broth

2 tbsp of olive oil

Preparation:

Wash the meat under cold running water and pat dry with a kitchen paper. Cut into bite-sized pieces. Set aside.

Place the rice in a deep pot and add 3 cups of water. Bring it to a boil and then reduce the heat to low. Cook for 15 minutes and remove from the heat.

Heat up the oil in a large skillet over a medium-high temperature. Add chicken chops and cook for 3 minutes, stirring occasionally. Add bell pepper and pour in the broth. Sprinkle with parsley and pepper. Stir well and bring it to a boil.

Stir in the rice and reduce the heat to low. Sprinkle with turmeric and give it a good final stir. Cook for 1-2 minutes more and remove from the heat.

Serve warm.

Nutrition information per serving: Kcal: 377, Protein: 30.6g, Carbs: 32.1g, Fats: 13.1g

11. Orange Ginger Smoothie

Ingredients:

2 large oranges, peeled and wedged

1 large green apple, cored and chopped

2 large peaches, pitted and chopped

½ cup of skim milk

1 tbsp of honey

¼ tsp of ginger, ground

Preparation:

Wash the apple and remove the core. Cut into bite-sized pieces and set aside.

Wash the peaches and cut in half. Remove the pits and chop it.

Peel the oranges and divide into wedges. Set aside.

Now, combine oranges, apple peaches, milk, honey, and ginger in a food processor. Blend until nicely smooth and creamy. Transfer to serving glasses and add some ice before serving.

Nutrition information per serving: Kcal: 129, Protein: 2.7g, Carbs: 31.4g, Fats: 0.4g

12.   Bell Pepper Soup

Ingredients:

1 large red bell pepper

1 large yellow bell pepper

1 large green bell pepper

2 cups of vegetable broth

1 cup of tomatoes, diced

1 large carrot, chopped

1 cup of broccoli, chopped

1 tsp of salt

¼ tsp of black pepper, ground

4 tbsp of tomato sauce

Preparation:

Wash the bell peppers and cut in half. Remove the seeds and cut into small slices. Wash the broccoli and cut into small pieces. Wash the carrot and cut into thin slices.

Now, combine all vegetables in a heavy-bottomed pot. Season with salt and pepper and pour the vegetable broth.

Bring it to a boil and then reduce the heat to low. Stir in the tomato sauce and cook for 30 minutes.

Remove from the heat and serve warm.

Nutrition information per serving: Kcal: 75, Protein: 4.7g, Carbs: 13.1g, Fats: 1.1g

13. Creamy Ziti Pasta

Ingredients:

1 lb of ziti pasta

1 large egg, beaten

1 small onion, chopped

2 garlic cloves, crushed

1 tbsp of lemon juice

2 tbsp of fresh parsley, finely chopped

1 cup of sour cream

1 cup of Cheddar cheese, shredded

Preparation:

Preheat the oven to 350°F.

Cook the pasta using package instructions. Drain well and set aside.

In a medium bowl, combine egg, onion, garlic, lemon juice, parsley, sour cream, cheese, and salt. Whisk with a kitchen hand mixer until well incorporated.

Grease a medium baking sheet with some oil and spread the pasta evenly on the bottom. Pour over the sour cream mixture and place it in the oven.

Bake for about 15 minutes, or until cheese gets bubbly. Remove from the oven and set aside to cool for a while before cutting and serving.

Nutrition information per serving: Kcal: 592, Protein: 23.6g, Carbs: 67.3g, Fats: 25.3g

14.   Fig Pancakes

Ingredients:

1 cup of all-purpose flour

2 large eggs

1 tbsp of liquid honey

1 tsp of baking powder

1 cup of skim milk

½ cup of fresh figs

½ cup of sour cream

2 tbsp of oil

Preparation:

Combine flour and baking powder in a medium bowl. Stir once and set aside.

In a separate bowl, whisk the eggs, honey, and milk. Stir in this mixture to a flour mixture with a hand mixer. Blend until you get a nice batter.

Now, grease a pancake pan with some oil. Heat up well to medium-high temperature. Pour about 1-2 tablespoons of pancake mixture into the pan.

Fry for about 1 minute on each side, or until lightly browned. Transfer to a plate and repeat the process with the remaining batter.

Combine figs, honey, and sour cream in a food processor. Blend until nicely smooth and transfer to a medium bowl.

Spoon the fig mixture to a pancake and roll them. Serve immediately.

Nutrition information per serving: Kcal: 373, Protein: 10.1g, Carbs: 49.1g, Fats: 15.9g

15.   Black Bean Potato Stew

Ingredients:

1 cup of black beans, soaked overnight

1 cup of tomatoes, diced

1 cup of sweet potatoes, cubed

3 garlic cloves

¼ cup of celery, finely chopped

2 small red onions, diced

1 tsp of salt

¼ tsp of red pepper flakes

3 cups of chicken broth

Preparation:

Soak the beans overnight. Drain and rinse well. Place the beans in a pot of boiling water and cook for 10 minutes. Remove from the heat and drain. Set aside.

In a heavy-bottomed pot, heat up the oil over a medium-high temperature. Add garlic and onions and stir-fry for 5 minutes. Add beans, tomatoes, sweet potatoes, celery, and broth. Sprinkle with salt and pepper and stir well. Reduce the heat to low and cover with a lid. Cook for 20 minutes, or until potatoes tender. Remove from the heat and serve warm

Nutrition information per serving: Kcal: 177, Protein: 10.4g, Carbs: 31.6g, Fats: 1.3g

16.   Grilled Sea Bream with Peppers

Ingredients:

2 lbs of sea bream fillets

1 tbsp of fresh rosemary, roughly chopped

1 cup of extra-virgin olive oil

1 tsp of sea salt

½ tsp of black pepper, freshly ground

2 garlic cloves, crushed

2 large red bell peppers, seeded and halved

Preparation:

Wash the fish fillets under cold running water and pat dry with a kitchen paper. Set aside.

In a large bowl, combine rosemary, oil, salt, pepper, and garlic. Stir until well incorporated. Soak the fish and peppers in this marinade and refrigerate for at least 30 minutes.

Preheat the grill to a medium-high temperature. Slightly drain the fillets and place on a grill. Fry for 3-5 minutes on each side, or until desired doneness.

Place the peppers on a grill and fry for 2 minutes on each side. Brush fillets and peppers with marinade from time to time.

Serve fish and peppers with boiled sweet potatoes or sour cream. However, this is optional.

Nutrition information per serving: Kcal: 436, Protein: 48.9g, Carbs: 4.6g, Fats: 24g

17.   Peach Oatmeal

Ingredients:

1 cup of rolled oats

1 cup of milk

1 large peach, pitted and chopped

1 tbsp of almonds, roughly chopped

1 tsp of vanilla extract

1 tbsp of agave syrup

Preparation:

Wash the peach and cut in half. Remove the pit and cut into bite-sized pieces. set aside.

Combine milk and oats in a deep pot over a medium-high temperature. Bring it to a boil and then reduce the heat to low. Cook for 5 minutes and then remove from the heat. Set aside to cool completely.

Stir in the peach, vanilla extract, and agave syrup. Top with almonds and serve immediately.

Nutrition information per serving: Kcal: 301, Protein: 10.7g, Carbs: 50g, Fats: 6.9g

18.   Avocado Risotto

Ingredients:

1 medium-sized avocado, peeled, pitted, cut into bite-sized pieces

1 cup of brown rice, pre-cooked

1 small onion, chopped

1 tbsp of olive oil

4 tbsp of chicken broth

¼ tsp of salt

¼ tsp of red pepper flakes

¼ tsp of Italian seasoning mix

Preparation:

Peel the avocado and cut in half. Remove the pit and cut into bite-sized pieces. Set aside.

Pour about 3 cups of water in a heavy-bottomed pot and add salt. Bring it to a boil and then stir in the rice. Reduce the heat to low and cook for about 15 minutes, stirring occasionally. Remove from the heat and set aside to cool completely.

In a large saucepan, heat up the oil over a medium-high temperature. Add onion and stir-fry for 3 minutes. Add avocado and reduce the heat to low. Pour the broth and cook for 5 minutes. Remove from the heat and set aside.

In a large bowl, combine rice with avocado and onion mixture. Sprinkle with red pepper and Italian seasoning mix. Stir all well and serve.

Nutrition information per serving: Kcal: 419, Protein: 6.7g, Carbs: 56.3g, Fats: 19.6g

19.   Creamy Veal Meatballs

Ingredients:

1 lb of lean veal, minced

½ cup of Gouda cheese, shredded

2 large eggs

3 tbsp of all-purpose flour

3 garlic cloves, crushed

1 tbsp of rosemary, finely chopped

½ tsp of salt

½ tsp of black pepper, ground

1 cup of sour cream

1 tbsp of fresh parsley, finely chopped

1 cup of chicken broth

Preparation:

Combine meat, cheese, eggs, flour, garlic, rosemary, salt, and pepper in a large bowl. Stir until well incorporated.

Combine sour cream and parsley in a small bowl. Stir well and set aside.

Grease a large heavy-bottomed pot with some cooking spray. Place the meatballs and fry for 5 minutes. Add chicken broth and bring it to a boil. Cook for 4 minutes, turning occasionally. Remove from the heat and transfer to a serving plate.

Pour the sour cream over the meatballs and serve.

Enjoy!

Nutrition information per serving: Kcal: 370, Protein: 31.7g, Carbs: 7.4g, Fats: 23.3g

20. Scrambled Eggs with Eggplant

Ingredients:

5 large eggs

½ cup of eggplant, chopped

1 small onion, chopped

¼ tsp of black pepper

1 tbsp of fresh parsley, finely chopped

1 tsp of salt

1 tbsp of olive oil

Preparation:

Wash and peel the eggplant. Cut into bite-sized pieces and fill the measuring cup. Sprinkle and coat with salt. This will reduce the bitterness of the eggplant. Reserve the rest in the refrigerator.

Preheat the oil in a large saucepan over a medium-sized temperature. Add eggplant and cook for about 3-4 minutes. Now, add onion and cook until onions translucent.

Crack the eggs and add directly to the vegetables. Stir with a wooden spatula and sprinkle with parsley and pepper. Cook until eggs are set and remove from the heat.

Serve immediately.

Nutrition information per serving: Kcal: 259, Protein: 16.4g, Carbs: 5.7g, Fats: 19.5g

21.   Turkey with Sun-Dried Tomatoes

Ingredients:

1 lb of turkey breasts, cut into bite-sized pieces

1 cup of sun-dried tomatoes,

1 small onion, finely chopped

2 garlic cloves, minced

2 cups of water

2 cups of chicken broth

1 tsp of salt

¼ tsp of black pepper, freshly ground

½ tsp of dried oregano, ground

1 tbsp of fresh basil, finely chopped

1 tbsp of olive oil

Preparation:

Wash the meat under cold running water and pat dry with a kitchen paper. Cut into bite-sized pieces and set aside.

Preheat the oil in a slow cooker over a medium-high temperature. Add onions and garlic and stir-fry for 4 minutes, or until translucent.

Add turkey chops and continue to cook until slightly browned, stirring occasionally.

Now, pour in the water and broth and season with oregano, basil, salt, and pepper. Reduce the heat to low and cook for 1 hour. Stir in the tomatoes and continue to cook for about 8 hours more on a low heat.

Remove from the heat and serve warm.

Nutrition information per serving: Kcal: 124, Protein: 15g, Carbs: 6.2g, Fats: 4.1g

22.   Spinach Potato Cream Soup

Ingredients:

1 lb of fresh spinach, chopped

2 medium-sized potatoes, chopped

3 tbsp of fresh parsley, chopped

1 small onion, finely chopped

2 tbsp of olive oil

2 tbsp of all-purpose flour

2 cups of chicken broth

1 cup of cream cheese

½ tsp of cayenne pepper

1 tsp of salt

¼ tsp of black pepper, ground

Preparation:

Wash and prepare the vegetables.

Place the spinach in a pot of boiling water and cook for 3 minutes, or until tender. Remove from the heat and drain. Set aside.

Place the potatoes in a pot of boiling water and sprinkle with some salt. Bring it to a boil and cook for 10minutes. Remove from the heat and drain. Set aside.

Preheat the oil in a large skillet over a medium-high temperature. Add onion and stir-fry until translucent. Stir in the flour, cayenne pepper, and 1 tablespoon of water. Cook for 1 minute, stirring constantly. Remove from the heat.

In a large heavy-bottomed pot, pour chicken broth and 1 cup of water. Bring it to a boil over a medium-high temperature. Add spinach and potatoes and sprinkle with pepper. Cook for 10 minutes, and reduce heat to low. Cook for another 5 minutes and then stir in the sour cream and parsley. Add some water to adjust the thickness of the soup.

Stir in the flour mixture and cook for 1 minute. Remove from the heat and set aside to cool for a while before serving.

Nutrition information per serving: Kcal: 231, Protein: 7.2g, Carbs: 15.9g, Fats: 16.3g

23.   Veal Steaks with Cranberry Sauce

Ingredients:

1 lb of veal steak

1 cup of olive oil

1 tsp of dried thyme, finely chopped

1 cup of rice, pre-cooked

½ cup of cranberries

1 tbsp of lemon juice, freshly squeezed

1 tsp of sea salt

1 small carrot, grated

1 cup of beef broth

½ tsp of black pepper, freshly ground

1 tsp of fresh rosemary, finely chopped

Preparation:

In a large bowl, combine oil, thyme, rosemary, salt, and pepper. Stir until well incorporated and soak the steaks. Refrigerate for 30 minutes.

Combine rice and carrot in a heavy-bottomed pot. Add beef broth and 1 cup of water. Bring it to a boil and then reduce the heat to low. Add a pinch of salt and cook for 15 minutes, stirring occasionally. Remove from the heat and set aside.

Now, preheat the grill to a medium-high temperature. Add steaks and grill for about 5 minutes on each side, or desired doneness. Generously brush the steaks with the marinade to get a more juicy steak. Remove from the heat and set aside.

Combine cranberries and lemon juice in a medium skillet over a medium-high temperature. Add ½ cup of water and bring it to a boil. Reduce the heat to low and stir occasionally until the mixture thickens. Remove from the heat.

Serve steaks with rice and pour over the cranberry sauce.

Enjoy!

Nutrition information per serving: Kcal: 362, Protein: 27.6g, Carbs: 32.2g, Fats: 12.5g

24.   Spinach Banana Smoothie

Ingredients:

1 large banana

1 cup of spinach, torn

1 tbsp of honey

1 cup of almond yogurt

1 tbsp of Brazil nuts, finely chopped

Preparation:

Wash the spinach thoroughly under cold running water. Drain and torn with hands. Set aside.

Peel the banana and cut into small chunks. Set aside.

Now, combine spinach, banana, honey, and yogurt in a food processor or a blender. Process until well smooth and transfer to serving glasses.

Top with nuts and refrigerate for 20 minutes before serving.

Nutrition information per serving: Kcal: 369, Protein: 12.3g, Carbs: 36.8g, Fats: 20.8g

25.   Chicken Fillets with Cayenne Sauce

Ingredients:

1 lb of chicken fillets, cut into bite-sized pieces

1 cup of broccoli, chopped

1 tbsp of butter

2 garlic cloves, minced

2 tbsp of lemon juice, freshly squeezed

2 tbsp of olive oil

1 tsp of salt

¼ tsp of black pepper, ground

2 tbsp of all-purpose flour

1 tsp of cayenne pepper

Preparation:

Wash the meat under cold running water and pat dry with a kitchen paper. Set aside.

Melt the butter in a large skillet over a medium-high temperature. Add broccoli and cook for 5 minutes, stirring occasionally. Remove from the heat and set aside.

Meanwhile, in a small pan, combine flour, cayenne pepper, salt, pepper, lemon juice, and 2 tablespoons of water. Stir well and cook for 2 minutes on low heat. Set aside.

Now, preheat the oil in a large frying pan over a medium-high temperature. Add garlic and stir-fry for 3-4 minutes, or until translucent. Add meat chops and cook for 5 minutes, stirring occasionally. Stir in the broccoli and pour over the cayenne pepper mixture. Stir well and cook for 2 minutes, or until well incorporated.

Remove from the heat and set serve warm.

Nutrition information per serving: Kcal: 438, Protein: 45.5g, Carbs: 7.3g, Fats: 24.7g

26. Vanilla Raisin Cookies

Ingredients:

2 cups of all-purpose flour

1 tsp of baking soda

½ tsp of salt

2 tbsp of honey

1 cup of raisins

1 tsp of vanilla extract

2 large eggs

1 cup of butter, melted

Preparation:

Preheat the oven to 375°F. Place some baking paper on a baking sheet and set aside.

In a large bowl, combine flour, soda, and salt. Stir and set aside.

In a separate bowl, whisk the eggs along with honey, butter, and honey. Now, stir in this mixture into the flour mixture and add raisins. Using an electric hand mixer, whisk until you get a nice batter.

Shape the cookies using your hands, about 1-inch thick. Place the cookie balls onto a sheet and press with your palms to form cookie shapes.

Place it in the oven and bake for about 10-12 minutes, or until nice and crispy. Remove from the heat and let it cool completely.

Serve cold.

Nutrition information per serving: Kcal: 325, Protein: 4.5g, Carbs: 34.2g, Fats: 19.7g

27.   Zucchini Oatmeal

Ingredients:

1 cup of rolled oats

1 cup of zucchini, peeled and chopped

2 cups of skim milk

2 tbsp of almonds, roughly chopped

1 tbsp of honey

Preparation:

Wash the zucchini and peel it. Cut into bite-sized pieces and place it in a pot of boiling water. Cook for 5 minutes or until tender. Remove from the heat and drain well. Set aside to cool for a while.

Combine oats and milk in a fire-proof dish and place it in the microwave. Heat it up for 3 minutes and then remove from the microwave.

Stir in the zucchini and honey into the oatmeal. Top with almonds and serve immediately.

Nutrition information per serving: Kcal: 214, Protein: 10.2g, Carbs: 34.3g, Fats: 10.2g

28.   Fresh Tomato Pepper Salad

Ingredients:

2 medium-sized tomatoes, chopped

1 large yellow bell pepper, chopped

1 cup of celery, chopped

1 small red onion, sliced

1 small cucumber, sliced

2 tbsp of fresh parsley, finely chopped

3 tbsp of extra-virgin olive oil

1 tbsp of balsamic vinegar

½ tsp of Himalayan pink salt

¼ tsp of black pepper, ground

¼ tsp of red pepper flakes

Preparation:

In a small bowl, combine oil, parsley, vinegar, salt, and pepper. Stir until well incorporated and set aside.

Now, combine tomatoes, bell pepper, cucumber, celery, and onion in a large salad bowl. Drizzle with previously prepared dressing and toss well to coat all ingredients.

Refrigerate for 10 minutes before serving.

Nutrition information per serving: Kcal: 135, Protein: 1.8g, Carbs: 10g, Fats: 10.9g

29. Grilled and Marinated Lamb Steaks

Ingredients:

1 lb of lamb steaks

1 medium-sized onion

1 cup of lamb's lettuce

2 garlic cloves, crushed

2 tbsp of lemon juice, freshly squeezed

1 cup of olive oil

1 tsp of dried thyme, ground

2 tbsp of fresh parsley, finely chopped

Preparation:

Wash the meat under cold running water and pat dry with a kitchen paper. Set aside.

In a large bowl, combine oil, garlic, lemon, thyme, and parsley. Stir well and then soak the meat in it. Refrigerate for 30 minutes in the marinade to allow flavors to penetrate into the meat.

Preheat the grill to medium-high temperature. Slightly drain the lamb steaks and place them on a grill rack. Grill for 5-8 minutes on each side, or desired doneness. Brush the meat with marinade occasionally.

Serve the steaks with lamb's lettuce.

Nutrition information per serving: Kcal: 386, Protein: 43.3g, Carbs: 5.2g, Fats: 20.6g

30. Onion Tuna Spread

Ingredients:

1lb of tuna fillets

1 large red onion, sliced

1 tsp of cayenne pepper, ground

3 tbsp of extra-virgin olive oil

¼ tsp of black pepper

¼ tsp of sea salt

1 tsp of dried rosemary, finely chopped

1 large red bell pepper, stripped

Preparation:

Wash the tuna fillets under cold running water and pat dry with a kitchen paper. Cut into bite-size pieces and set aside.

Heat up the oil in a large skillet and add onions. Sprinkle with cayenne pepper and cook for about 3-4 minutes, or until translucent. Add tuna chops and cook for 4 minutes, stirring occasionally. Remove from the heat and set aside to cool for a while.

Now, combine tuna and onion mixture along with other ingredients in a blender. Process for 2 minutes, or until well blended.

Serve tuna spread with some fresh bell pepper strips.

Nutrition information per serving: Kcal: 263, Protein: 24.7g, Carbs: 5g, Fats: 15.9g

31. Chicken with Collard Greens

Ingredients:

1 lb of chicken fillets, cut into bite-sized pieces

1 cup of collard greens, chopped

3 tbsp of olive oil

1 tsp of dried thyme, ground

1 tsp of salt

¼ tsp of black pepper, freshly ground

Preparation:

Wash the meat under cold running water and pat dry with a kitchen paper. Cut into bite-sized pieces and set aside.

Wash the collard greens thoroughly and chop into small pieces. Place in a pot of boiling water and cook for 5 minutes. Remove from the heat and drain well. Set aside.

Now, preheat the oil in a large skillet over a medium-high temperature. Add chicken and sprinkle with thyme, salt, and pepper to taste. Cook for 10 minutes, stirring occasionally.

Reduce the heat to low and cook for 5 more minutes. Remove from the heat and serve warm.

Nutrition information per serving: Kcal: 413, Protein: 44.1g, Carbs: 1.2g, Fats: 25.3g

32. Almond Quinoa Porridge

Ingredients:

1 cup of quinoa

1 cup of water

1 tbsp of honey

1 cup of almond milk

2 tbsp of almonds, finely chopped

Preparation:

In a heavy-bottomed pot, combine quinoa and water. Bring it to a boil and then reduce the heat. Cover with a lid and cook for 15 minutes. Remove from the heat and drain the excessive liquid. Whisk with a fork and set aside.

Now, combine quinoa, milk, and honey in a clean pot. Cook until heated thoroughly and remove from the heat. Top with almonds and set aside to cool for a while.

Enjoy!

Nutrition information per serving: Kcal: 437, Protein: 10.7g, Carbs: 47.4g, Fats: 24.5g

33. Peanut Butter Balls

Ingredients:

1 ½ cup of rolled oats

3 cups of milk

½ cup of peanut butter

1 tbsp of vanilla extract

4 tbsp of almonds, minced

3 tbsp of honey

1 tbsp of chia seeds, minced

Preparation:

Place one cup of rolled oats in a bowl. Add other dry ingredients and stir to combine.

Now add in peanut butter and honey. Mix well and gently pour in the milk and vanilla extract. Shape the balls using your hands, top with the remaining oats and place in the refrigerator for about 30 minutes.

Nutrition information per serving: Kcal: 425, Protein: 31g, Carbs: 48g, Fats: 10.5g

34. Chicken Cauliflower Soup

Ingredients:

10 oz of chicken fillets, cut into bite-sized pieces

2 oz cauliflower, chopped

1 tsp of fresh mint, finely chopped

¼ tsp of dry coriander, crushed

1 tbsp of olive oil

½ tsp of salt

¼ tsp of black pepper

Preparation:

Place the cauliflower and dry coriander into a deep pot. Add enough water to cover and bring it to a boil. Cook for about 10-15 minutes. Remove from the heat and blend the soup with a stick blender. Set aside.

Now, preheat the oil in a large skillet over a medium-high temperature. Add meat chops and sprinkle with some salt and pepper. Cook for 5-8 minutes, or until golden brown. Remove from the heat and add it to the soup.

Reheat the soup and garnish with fresh mint before serving.

Nutrition information per serving: Kcal: 338, Protein: 41.6g, Carbs: 1.8g, Fats: 17.6g

35. Mediterranean Mackerel

Ingredients:

2 lbs of fresh mackerel

2 tbsp of extra-virgin olive oil

1 large lemon, sliced

1 tbsp of dry mint, ground

3 garlic cloves, crushed

¼ tsp of red pepper flakes

1 tsp of sea salt

1 tbsp of fresh rosemary, finely chopped

Preparation:

Cut the fish lengthwise and remove entrails. Wash it thoroughly under cold running water and pat dry with a kitchen paper. Set aside.

Combine the olive oil with dry mint, crushed garlic cloves, and red pepper. Brush the fish with this mixture and stuff with lemon slices and rosemary.

Preheat the electric grill to a medium-high temperature. Fry for about 5-7 minutes on each side.

Serve the fish with cooked potatoes or steamed spinach.

Nutrition information per serving: Kcal: 533, Protein: 43.6g, Carbs: 2.3g, Fats: 38.1g

36.   Mushroom Cheese Patties

Ingredients:

1 cup of button mushrooms, chopped

1 medium-sized sweet potato, peeled and cubed

1 cup of fresh spinach, chopped

½ cup of brown rice

1 cup of Cheddar cheese, crumbled

3 large egg whites

½ cup of chia seeds

2 cups of bread crumbs

1 tsp of tarragon

1 tsp of fresh parsley, finely chopped

1 garlic clove, crushed

Preparation:

Pour 2 cups of water in a small saucepan. Bring it to a boil and then add rice. Cook for about 10 minutes, until slightly sticky.

Meanwhile, combine chia seeds with 1 cup of water in a separate pot. Bring it to a boil and then cook 3 minutes, until soften. Remove from the heat and set aside.

Wash and finely chop the mushrooms. Thoroughly rinse spinach and chop it.

Now, combine rice, chia, mushrooms, spinach, and remaining ingredients. Stir well until nice dough forms. Refrigerate it for 30 minutes.

Take mixture out of the fridge and form into patties. Make sure cooking surfaces are cleaned and greased before adding patties to prevent them from sticking.

Grease a large frying pan with a cooking spray. Fry each piece for about 5 minutes on each side, or the desired doneness. Remove from the heat and serve with sour cream or fresh vegetable salad.

Nutrition information per serving: Kcal: 449, Protein: 24.g, Carbs: 76.8g, Fats: 14.7g

37.   Cranberry Pancakes with Almond Cream

Ingredients:

1 cup of fresh cranberries

1 cup of almond cream

1 cup of almond milk

12 tbsp of water

4 tbsp of buckwheat flour

¼ tsp of salt

1 tbsp coconut oil

4 tbsp of flax seed

Preparation:

In a small bowl, combine 4 tablespoons of flax seed with 12 tablespoons of water. Set aside

Combine other ingredients in a bowl and add flax seed mixture. Beat well with an electric mixer, on high.

Melt the oil in a medium-sized skillet, over a medium-high temperature. Pour some of the mixture in the skillet and fry the pancakes for about 2-3 minutes, on each side. This mixture should give you about 8 pancakes.

Top each pancake with almond cream and fresh cranberries.

Serve immediately.

Nutrition information per serving: Kcal: 373, Protein: 5.7g, Carbs: 18.3g, Fats: 32.3g

38.   Black and Green Beans Salad

Ingredients:

1 cup of black beans, soaked overnight

1 cup of green beans, chopped

½ cup of fresh celery, chopped

½ cup of Mozzarella cheese, crumbled

2 tbsp of fresh parsley, finely chopped

1 tsp of cayenne pepper, ground

¼ tsp of dried oregano, ground

1 tsp of salt

2 tbsp of lemon juice, freshly squeezed

3 tbsp of olive oil

Preparation:

Soak the black beans overnight. Rinse under cold running water and place in a deep pot. Add about 2 cups of water and bring it to a boil. Reduce the heat to low and cover with a lid. Cook for 30 minutes, or until tender. Remove from the heat and drain well. Set aside.

Wash the green beans under cold running water and drain well. Cut into bite-sized pieces and set aside.

Wash the celery and cut into bite-sized pieces. Set aside.

In a small bowl, combine 2 tablespoons of olive oil, lemon juice, parsley, salt, oregano, and cayenne pepper. Stir well and set aside for 10 minutes to allow flavors to meld.

Preheat the remaining oil in a large skillet over a medium-high temperature. Add green beans and cook for 10 minutes, stirring occasionally.

In a large bowl, combine black beans, green beans, cheese, and celery. Stir to combine and drizzle with the previously made dressing. Toss well to coat all ingredients and refrigerate for 15 minutes before serving.

Nutrition information per serving: Kcal: 374, Protein: 16.3g, Carbs: 44.4g, Fats: 16g

39.   Rosemary Turkey Chops

Ingredients:

1 lb of turkey fillets

3 tbsp of lemon juice, freshly squeezed

1 tbsp of extra-virgin olive oil

1 tbsp of butter

2 garlic cloves, crushed

1 tbsp of fresh rosemary, finely chopped

1 tsp of salt

¼ tsp of black pepper, freshly ground

Preparation:

Wash the fillets under cold running water and pat dry with a kitchen paper. Cut into bite-sized pieces and set aside.

In a medium bowl, combine lemon juice, olive oil, rosemary, salt, and pepper. Stir until well incorporated and set aside.

Melt the butter in a large saucepan over a medium-high temperature. Add meat chops and cook for 5 minutes, or until golden brown. Drizzle with previously prepared sauce and cook for 1 minute more.

Remove from the heat and serve immediately.

Nutrition information per serving: Kcal: 342, Protein: 44.6g, Carbs: 1.8g, Fats: 16.4g

40.   Shrimps in Lemon Sauce

Ingredients:

1 lb of fresh shrimps, peeled and deveined

½ cup of lemon, freshly squeezed

1 tsp of salt

2 tbsp of extra-virgin olive oil

¼ tsp of black pepper, ground

¼ tsp of red pepper flakes

1 tbsp of fresh parsley, finely chopped

1 tbsp of fresh rosemary, finely chopped

Preparation:

In a small bowl, combine lemon, salt, pepper, red pepper, parsley, and rosemary. Stir until well incorporated and set aside.

Preheat the oil in a large skillet over a medium to high temperature. Cook for about 5-7 minutes, or until almost done. Drizzle over the marinade and cook for 1 minute more. Remove from the heat and serve immediately.

Nutrition information per serving: Kcal: 275, Protein: 35g, Carbs: 6.6g, Fats: 12.2g

41.   Portobello Mushrooms

Ingredients:

6 Portobello mushrooms

6 oz of smoked salmon, finely chopped

6 large eggs, beaten

1 cup of cheddar cheese

1 tsp of fresh rosemary, finely chopped

3 tbsp of olive oil

½ tsp of sea salt

¼ tsp of black pepper, ground

Preparation:

Wash the mushrooms and remove the caps. Scrape out the flesh and make bowl-like shapes. Set aside.

In a medium bowl, combine cheese, eggs, salmon, rosemary, salt, and pepper.

Preheat 1 tablespoon of olive oil in a large frying pan over a medium-high temperature. Use the remaining oil to brush the mushrooms.

Cook the mushrooms for about 3-4 minutes, reduce the heat to low and cook for 5 more minutes. Remove from the heat and serve immediately.

Nutrition information per serving: Kcal: 308, Protein: 22.1g, Carbs: 3.8g, Fats: 23.6g

42. Cutlets with Bell Peppers

Ingredients:

1 lb of lamb cutlets

1 medium-sized green pepper, chopped

1 medium-sized yellow pepper, chopped

1 medium-sized tomato, chopped

1 small onion, chopped

1 cup of olive oil

1 tsp of salt

¼ tsp of black pepper, ground

4 tbsp of lemon juice, freshly squeezed

2 tbsp balsamic vinegar

Preparation:

Wash the meat under cold running water and pat dry with a kitchen paper. Set aside.

In a large bowl, combine olive oil, vinegar, salt, pepper, and lemon juice. Stir well and soak the meat in this marinade. Refrigerate for 20 minutes.

Now, use about 2 tablespoons of the marinade and heat up in a large frying pan over a medium-high temperature. Add cutlets and cook for about 12-15 minutes, or until desired doneness. You can add some more marinade while cooking to get it juicier and cooked evenly. Remove from the heat and transfer to a serving plate. Add washed and prepared vegetables and serve immediately.

Nutrition information per serving: Kcal: 453, Protein: 22.1g, Carbs: 5.1g, Fats: 39.4g

43.   Oven-Baked Thighs with Cashews

Ingredients:

1 lb of chicken thighs, skinless and boneless

3 tbsp of cashews, finely chopped

1 medium-sized red onion, sliced

1 large sweet potatoes, peeled and cubed

1 small red bell pepper, sliced

1 tbsp of fresh parsley, finely chopped

2 garlic cloves, crushed

2 tbsp of olive oil

1 tsp of salt

¼ tsp of black pepper, ground

Preparation:

Preheat the oven to 325°F.

Wash the chicken thighs under cold running water and pat dry with a kitchen paper. Set aside.

In a small bowl, combine cashews, oil, parsley, garlic, salt, and pepper. Stir until well incorporated and set aside.

Now, combine chicken thighs, onion, potatoes, and bell pepper on a large baking sheet. Drizzle with previously prepared sauce and place it in the oven.

Bake for about 30-35 minutes, or until set. Remove from the oven and let it cool for a while.

Nutrition information per serving: Kcal: 221, Protein: 35.1g, Carbs: 18g, Fats: 18.6g

44.   Creamy Eggs with Cherry Tomatoes

Ingredients:

5 large eggs, beaten

1 small onion, finely chopped

½ cup of cherry tomatoes, diced

2 tbsp of skim milk

1 tbsp of cream cheese

½ tsp of dried oregano, ground

1 tbsp of olive oil

½ tsp of salt

Preparation:

In a large bowl, whisk the eggs, milk, and cream cheese with a hand mixer for 2 minutes, or until well combined.

Preheat the olive oil in a large nonstick saucepan over a medium-high temperature. Add onions and stir-fry for 2 minutes then add diced tomatoes. Cook for another 2 minutes and pour the egg mixture. Sprinkle with oregano and cook until the eggs are set. Remove from the heat and serve immediately.

Nutrition information per serving: Kcal: 285, Protein: 17.4g, Carbs: 7.1g, Fats: 21.3g

45.　Grill Marinated Tuna Steaks

Ingredients:

1 lb of tuna steaks, skinless and boneless

4 tbsp of lemon juice, freshly squeezed

1 cup of olive oil

2 tbsp of fresh rosemary, finely chopped

1 tbsp of fresh parsley, finely chopped

3 garlic cloves, crushed

1 tsp of sea salt

¼ tsp of black pepper, freshly ground

Preparation:

Wash the steaks under cold running water and pat dry with a kitchen paper. Set aside.

In a large bowl combine lemon juice, rosemary, parsley, garlic, salt, and pepper. Stir well and soak the steaks in this marinade. Refrigerate for 20 minutes before cooking.

Preheat the grill to a medium-high temperature. Grill the steaks for about 5-6 minutes on each side.

Remove from the grill and serve immediately.

Nutrition information per serving: Kcal: 416, Protein: 45.7g, Carbs: 3g, Fats: 24g

46.   Roasted Pecans and Arugula Salad

Ingredients:

1 lb of fresh arugula, chopped

1 large apple, pitted and wedged

2 tbsp of lemon juice, freshly squeezed

1 small onion, sliced

2 tbsp of extra-virgin olive oil

2 oz of pecans, roughly chopped

1 tbsp of liquid honey

1 tsp of sea salt

¼ tsp of black pepper, freshly ground

Preparation:

Preheat the oven to 300°F.

Place a small piece of baking paper on a small baking sheet and place the nuts onto it. Place it in the oven and bake for 10 minutes, or until golden brown. Remove from the oven and set aside to cool for a while.

In a small bowl, combine lemon juice, oil, honey, salt, and

pepper. Stir until well incorporated and set aside to allow flavors to meld.

Wash the arugula thoroughly under cold running water. Drain and roughly chop it in a large salad bowl. Set aside.

Wash the apple and cut in half. Remove the core and slice the apple into wedges. Add it to the bowl with arugula and set aside.

Peel the onion and slice into thin slices. Add it to the bowl with other ingredients.

Now, drizzle the salad with dressing and toss well to coat all the ingredients. Top with roasted pecans and serve immediately.

Nutrition information per serving: Kcal: 241, Protein: 4.9g, Carbs: 20.1g, Fats: 18g

47.   Curry Turkey Stew

Ingredients:

1 lb of turkey fillets, cut into bite-sized pieces

1 tbsp of curry, ground

½ cup of scallions, finely chopped

2 garlic cloves, minced

2 medium-sized carrots, sliced

3 cups of chicken broth

1 tsp of salt

½ tsp of black pepper, freshly ground

1 tbsp of lime juice

2 tbsp of olive oil

Preparation:

Wash the meat under cold running water and pat dry with a kitchen paper. Cut into bite-sized pieces and set aside.

Preheat the oil in a large nonstick saucepan over a medium-high temperature. Add garlic, scallions, carrots, and ginger and cook for 3 minutes, stirring occasionally. Now, add turkey and cook for about 3-4 minutes, or until slightly brown.

Pour in the broth and sprinkle with salt and pepper. Bring it to a boil and then reduce the heat to low. Cook for 15 minutes and remove from the heat.

Sprinkle with lime juice before serving.

Nutrition information per serving: Kcal: 205, Protein: 25.1g, Carbs: 4.2g, Fats: 9.3g

48.   Grilled Sweet Trout

Ingredients:

1 lb of trout fillets

1 small onion, finely chopped

2 tbsp of lemon juice, freshly squeezed

½ cup of olive oil

1 tbsp of agave syrup

2 tbsp of orange juice, freshly squeezed

1 tsp of dried rosemary, ground

1 tsp of salt

½ tsp of black pepper, freshly ground

Preparation:

Wash the fish fillets under cold running water and pat dry with a kitchen paper. Set aside.

In a large bowl, combine onions, lemon juice, orange juice, oil, agave, rosemary, salt and pepper. Stir until well incorporated and soak the fish fillets in this marinade. Refrigerate for 30 minutes to allow flavors to penetrate into the fish.

Preheat a large grilling pan over a medium-high temperature. Add marinated fish fillets and grill for about 4-5 minutes on each side.

Transfer to a serving plate and drizzle with more marinade.

Nutrition information per serving: Kcal: 407, Protein: 40.7g, Carbs: 9.6g, Fats: 22.3g

49.   Artichoke Beet Smoothie

Ingredients:

1 medium-sized artichoke, chopped

1 cup of beets, trimmed and chopped

1 cup of Greek yogurt

½ tsp of turmeric, ground

1 large cucumber

Preparation:

Trim off the artichoke and cut into bite-sized pieces. Fill the measuring cup and reserve the rest in a refrigerator. Set aside.

Wash the beets and trim off the green parts. Cut into bite-sized pieces and set aside.

Wash the cucumber and cut into thick slices. Set aside.

Combine artichoke, beets, yogurt, turmeric, and cucumber in a food processor. Blend until nicely smooth and transfer to serving glasses.

Refrigerate for 20 minutes before serving.

Nutrition information per serving: Kcal: 93, Protein: 8.6g, Carbs: 13g, Fats: 1.5g

50.   Apple Coconut Oatmeal

Ingredients:

1 cup of rolled oats

1 small Honey Crisp apple, cored and grated

2 tbsp of honey

1 cup of coconut milk

1 tbsp of fresh mint, finely chopped

Preparation:

Combine oats and coconut milk in a heavy-bottomed pot over a low temperature. Cook for 2 minutes, or until heated completely. Do not boil.

Remove from the heat and stir in the grated apple and honey. Sprinkle with fresh mint a set aside to cool completely before serving.

Enjoy!

Nutrition information per serving: Kcal: 554, Protein: 8.6g, Carbs: 67.3g, Fats: 31.5g

51.   Rosemary Meatballs

Ingredients:

1 lb of lean beef, minced

1 small onion, chopped

1 tbsp of fresh rosemary, finely chopped

1 large egg

2 tbsp of all-purpose flour

1 tbsp of olive oil

½ tsp of salt

¼ tsp of black pepper, ground

¼ tsp of red pepper flakes

Preparation:

In a large bowl, combine all ingredients and mix with your hands until all well incorporated.

Shape the meatballs into the desired size and set aside.

Preheat the oil in a large skillet over a medium-high temperature. Add meatballs and cook for about 10 minutes, turning occasionally. Remove from the heat when lightly charred.

Serve with sour cream, yogurt, or fresh salad.

Enjoy!

Nutrition information per serving: Kcal: 378, Protein: 48.9g, Carbs: 7.2g, Fats: 16g

52.   Marinated Chicken with Mustard

Ingredients:

2 lbs of chicken breasts, skinless and boneless

1 cup of olive oil

2 tbsp of apple cider vinegar

2 garlic cloves, crushed

2 tbsp of Dijon mustard

2 tbsp of fresh parsley, finely chopped

1 tsp of salt

¼ tsp of black pepper, freshly ground

Preparation:

Wash the meat under cold running water and pat dry with a kitchen paper. Gently rub with a salt and pepper and place on a cutting board. Cut into bite-sized pieces and set aside.

In a large bowl, combine olive oil, vinegar, garlic, mustard, and parsley. Stir until well incorporated. Soak the meat chops in this marinade for at least to 2 hours.

Use one tablespoon of the marinade and pour it into a large saucepan. Heat it up to a medium-high temperature. Add meat chops and cook for 8-10 minutes, or until golden brown and crisp. Add more marinade while cooking to get it juicier.

Remove from the heat and serve warm.

Nutrition information per serving: Kcal: 449, Protein: 52.9g, Carbs: 1g, Fats: 24.9g

JUICES

1.   Cucumber Radish Juice

Ingredients:

1 large cucumber, sliced

3 large radishes, trimmed

2 cups of beets, trimmed

1 large Roma tomato, chopped

½ tsp of fresh rosemary, chopped

¼ tsp of sea salt

1 oz of water

Preparation:

Wash the cucumber and cut into thin slices. Set aside.

Wash the radishes and trim off the green ends. Cut in half and set aside.

Wash the beets and trim off the green parts. Cut into small pieces and set aside.

Wash the tomato and place it in a bowl. Cut into bite-sized pieces and reserve the tomato juice while cutting. Set aside.

Now, combine, cucumber, radishes, beets, tomato, and rosemary in a juicer. Process until well juiced and transfer to serving glasses. Stir in the salt and water. Refrigerate for 5 minutes before serving.

Enjoy!

Nutritional information per serving: Kcal: 152, Protein: 8.2g, Carbs: 44.9g, Fats: 1.2g

2.   Apricot Cantaloupe Juice

Ingredients:

1 cup of apricots, pitted and halved

1 cup of cantaloupe, chopped

2 large peaches, pitted and halved

3 oz of coconut water

Preparation:

Wash the apricots and cut in half. Remove the pits and fill the measuring cup. Reserve the rest for some other juice. Set aside.

Cut the cantaloupe in half. Scoop out the seeds and cut about two large wedges. Peel and chop into chunks. Fill the measuring cup and reserve the rest of the cantaloupe in a refrigerator for some other juice.

Wash the peaches and cut in half. Remove the pits and cut into bite-sized pieces. Set aside.

Now, process apricots, cantaloupe, and peaches in a juicer.

Transfer to serving glasses and stir in the coconut water. Add some ice and serve immediately.

Nutrition information per serving: Kcal: 239, Protein: 6.8g, Carbs: 66.4g, Fats: 1.8g

3.   Carrot Watercress Juice

Ingredients:

2 large carrots

½ cup of watercress

1 cup of pineapple, peeled

1 large lemon, peeled

¼ tsp of ginger root

Preparation:

Wash the carros and cut into small pieces. Set aside.

Wash the watercress thoroughly under cold running water. Drain and roughly chop it into small pieces. Set aside.

Peel the pineapple and cut into small chunks. Set aside.

Peel the lemon and cut into quarters. Set aside.

Peel the ginger root slice and cut into halves.

Process pineapple, then carrots, watercress, lemon, and ginger root. Transfer to serving glasses and a little bit of water to adjust the thickness of the juice. Add some ice and serve.

Nutritional information per serving: Kcal: 101, Protein: 3.1g, Carbs: 34.2g, Fats: 1.1g

4.   Blueberry Lime Juice

Ingredients:

1 cup of blueberries

1 whole lime, peeled

1 cup of pomegranate seeds

1 small Granny Smith's apple, cored

¼ tsp of ginger, ground

2 oz of water

Preparation:

Place the blueberries in a colander. Rinse well under cold running water and drain. Set aside.

Peel the lime and cut lengthwise in half. Set aside.

Cut the top of the pomegranate fruit using a sharp paring knife. Slice down to each of the white membranes inside of the fruit. Pop the seeds into a measuring cup and set aside.

Wash the apple and cut lengthwise in half. Remove the core and cut into bite-sized pieces and set aside.

Now, combine pomegranate seeds, blueberries, lime, and apple in a juicer and process until juiced. Transfer to a serving glass and stir in the ginger and water.

Refrigerate for 10 minutes before serving.

Enjoy!

Nutritional information per serving: Kcal: 206, Protein: 3.3g, Carbs: 61.1g, Fats: 1.8g

5.   Celery Watercress Juice

Ingredients:

1 cup of celery, chopped

1 cup of watercress, chopped

2 cups of beets, trimmed

1 cup of Romaine lettuce, chopped

1 cup of basil, chopped

A handful of spinach

¼ tsp of Himalayan salt

2 oz of water

Preparation:

Combine lettuce, celery, watercress, basil, and spinach in a colander. Wash thoroughly under cold running water and drain. Roughly chop and set aside.

Wash the beets and trim off the green parts. Cut into bite-sized pieces and set aside.

Now, process celery, watercress, basil, beets, lettuce, and spinach in a juicer.

Transfer to serving glasses and stir in the salt and water. Add few ice cubes before serving and enjoy!

Nutritional information per serving: Kcal: 111, Protein: 8.1g, Carbs: 32.7g, Fats: 1.1g

6.   Citrus Zucchini Juice

Ingredients:

1 large lemon, peeled

1 large lime, peeled

1 medium-sized zucchini, chopped

1 large artichoke, chopped

1 cup of fresh basil, chopped

1 cup of green cabbage, chopped

2 oz of water

Preparation:

Peel the lemon and lime. Cut lengthwise in half and set aside.

Peel the zucchini and cut lengthwise in half. Scoop out the seeds and peel it. Cut into bite-sized pieces and set aside.

Trim off the outer leaves of the artichoke. Wash it and cut into bite-sized pieces. Set aside.

Combine basil and cabbage in a colander. Wash thoroughly under cold running water and roughly chop it. Set aside.

Now, combine lemon, lime, zucchini, artichoke, basil, and cabbage in a juicer. Process until well juiced and stir in the water.

Refrigerate for 5 minutes before serving.

Enjoy!

Nutritional information per serving: Kcal: 104, Protein: 10.4g, Carbs: 38.1g, Fats: 1.3g

7. Beet Apricot Juice

Ingredients:

1 cup of beets, trimmed and sliced

1 cup of apricots, sliced

1 large peach, pitted and chopped

1 whole lemon, peeled and halved

1 small ginger slice, peeled

1 oz of water

Preparation:

Wash the beets and trim off the green ends. Slightly peel and cut into thin slices. Fill the measuring cup and reserve the rest for later.

Wash the apricots and cut lengthwise in half. Remove the pits and cut into thin slices. Fill the measuring cup and reserve the rest in the refrigerator.

Wash the peach and cut lengthwise in half. Remove the pit and chop into bite-sized pieces. Set aside.

Peel the ginger slice and chop into small pieces. Set aside.

Now, combine beets, apricots, peach, lemon, and ginger in a juicer and process until juiced. Transfer to a serving glass and stir in the water.

Refrigerate for 10 minutes, or add some ice before serving.

Nutritional information per serving: Kcal: 180, Protein: 6.7g, Carbs: 53.8g, Fats: 1.5g

8.   Apple Kale Juice

Ingredients:

1 large green apple, cored

1 cup of kale, torn

3 medium-sized radishes, trimmed

3 large leeks, chopped

1 large cucumber

A handful of fresh spinach, torn

Preparation:

Wash the apple and remove the core. Cut into bite-sized pieces and set aside.

Combine kale and spinach in a colander. Wash thoroughly under cold running water and torn with hands.

Wash the radishes and trim off the green ends. Cut into small pieces and set aside.

Wash the leeks and chop into small pieces. Set aside.

Wash the cucumber and cut into thick slices. Set aside.

Now, process apple, kale, radishes, leeks, cucumber, and spinach in a juicer. Transfer to serving glasses and add some ice before serving.

Enjoy!

Nutritional information per serving: Kcal: 315, Protein: 10.4g, Carbs: 85.3g, Fats: 2.2g

9.　　Kiwi Lime Juice

Ingredients:

1 large kiwi, peeled

1 large lime, peeled

2 large grapefruits, peeled

2 large celery stalks, chopped

1 cup of red leaf lettuce, chopped

2 oz of water

Preparation:

Peel the kiwi and lime. Cut in half and set aside.

Peel the grapefruit and divide into wedges. Set aside.

Wash and chop the celery stalks into small pieces. Set aside.

Wash the lettuce thoroughly under cold running water and roughly chop it. Set aside.

Now, combine kiwi, lime, grapefruit, celery, and lettuce in a juicer and process until well juiced.Transfer to serving glasses and stir in the water.

Serve immediately.

Nutritional information per serving: Kcal: 233, Protein: 6g, Carbs: 70.7g, Fats: 1.3g

10.   Orange Guava Juice

Ingredients:

2 large oranges, peeled

1 large guava, peeled

1 large lime, peeled

1 large cucumber, sliced

2 oz of water

Preparation:

Peel the oranges and divide into wedges. Set aside.

Peel and wash the guava. Cut into small chunks and set aside.

Peel the lime and cut lengthwise in half. Set aside.

Wash the cucumber and cut into thin slices. Set aside.

Now, combine orange, guava, lime, orange, and cucumber in a juicer and process until juiced.

Transfer to serving glasses and stir in the water. Add some ice and serve immediately.

Nutritional information per serving: Kcal: 210, Protein: 7g, Carbs: 65.7g, Fats: 1.3g

11.   Pepper Lettuce Juice

Ingredients:

1 large yellow bell pepper, chopped

1 cup of Romaine lettuce, chopped

1 cup of fennel, sliced

1 cup of cucumber, sliced

1 small zucchini, cubed

Preparation:

Wash the bell pepper and cut lengthwise in half. Remove the stem and seeds. Cut into small pieces and set aside.

Wash the Romaine lettuce thoroughly under cold running water. Drain and chop into small pieces. Set aside.

Trim off the fennel bulb and remove the green parts. Wash it and cut into small pieces. Fill the measuring cup and reserve the rest for later. Set aside.

Wash the cucumber and cut into thin slices. Fill the measuring cup and reserve the rest for later.

Wash the zucchini and cut into small cubes. Set aside.

Now, combine bell pepper, lettuce, fennel, cucumber, and zucchini in a juicer and process until juiced. Transfer to a serving glass and refrigerate for 10 minutes before serving.

Nutritional information per serving: Kcal: 85, Protein: 5.3g, Carbs: 25.2g, Fats: 1.1g

12. Cranberry Watermelon Juice

Ingredients:

1 cup of cranberries

1 cup of watermelon, seeded

1 cup of cantaloupe, chopped

1 large lemon, peeled

1 small Ginger Gold apple, cored

1 small ginger root slice

Preparation:

Wash the cranberries under cold running water using a colander. Drain and set aside.

Cut the watermelon lengthwise in half. For one cup, you will need about 1 large wedge. Peel and cut into chunks. Remove the seeds and set aside.

Cut the cantaloupe in half. Scoop out the seeds and flesh. Cut two wedges and peel them. Chop into chunks and fill the measuring cup. Reserve the rest of the cantaloupe in a refrigerator.

Peel the lemon and cut lengthwise in half. Set aside.

Wash the apple and remove the core. Cut into bite-sized pieces and set aside.

Peel the ginger root and set aside.

Now, combine cranberries, watermelon, cantaloupe, lemon, apple, and ginger in a juicer and process until juiced.

Transfer to serving glasses and refrigerate for 5 minutes before serving.

Nutritional information per serving: Kcal: 194, Protein: 3.6g, Carbs: 59.7g, Fats: 1.1g

13.　Squash Plum Juice

Ingredients:

1 cup of butternut squash, cubed

2 whole plums, pitted and chopped

1 cup of strawberries, chopped

1 medium-sized apple, cored

¼ tsp of ginger, ground

¼ tsp of turmeric, ground

Preparation:

Peel the butternut squash and cut lengthwise in half. Scoop out the seeds and wash the both halves. Cut into small cubes and fill the measuring cup. Wrap the rest of the squash in a plastic foil and refrigerate for later.

Wash the plums and cut in half. Remove the pits and cut into bite-sized pieces. Set aside.

Wash the strawberries and remove the stems. Cut into bite-sized pieces and fill the measuring cup. Reserve the rest in the refrigerator. Set aside.

Wash the apple and cut lengthwise in half. Remove the core and cut into bite-sized pieces. Set aside.

Now, combine butternut squash, plum, strawberries, and apple in a juicer and process until well juiced. Transfer to a serving glass and add some crushed ice.

Serve immediately.

Nutrition information per serving: Kcal: 214, Protein: 4.1g, Carbs: 65.2g, Fats: 1.2g

14.   Spinach Lemon Juice

Ingredients:

1 cup of fresh spinach, torn

1 whole lemon, peeled

1 medium-sized tomato, chopped

1 large red bell pepper, chopped

1 tsp of rosemary, finely chopped

Preparation:

Wash the spinach thoroughly under cold running water. Drain and torn into small pieces. Set aside.

Peel the lemon and cut lengthwise in half. Set aside.

Wash the tomato and place in a small bowl. Chop into small pieces and reserve the tomato juice while cutting. Set aside.

Wash the bell pepper and cut in half. Remove the stem and seeds. Cut into small pieces and set aside.

Now, combine spinach, lemon, tomato, and bell pepper in a juicer and process until juiced. Transfer to a serving glass and stir in the rosemary.

Add few ice cubes and serve immediately.

Nutritional information per serving: Kcal: 92, Protein: 9.3g, Carbs: 27.7g, Fats: 1.7g

15.   Beet Pepper Juice

Ingredients:

2 cups of beet greens

1 large red bell pepper, seeded

1 cup of cherry tomatoes

1 cup of celery, chopped

1 small rosemary sprig

Preparation:

Combine beet greens and celery in a colander and wash thoroughly under cold running water. Roughly chop it and set aside.

Wash the bell pepper and cut in half. Remove the seeds and chop into small pieces. Set aside.

Wash the cherry tomatoes and place them in a bowl. Cut in half and fill the measuring cup. Reserve the tomato juice while cutting. Set aside.

Now, combine beet greens, bell pepper, cherry tomatoes, and celery in a juicer and process until juiced.

Transfer to serving glasses and stir in the reserved tomato juice and sprinkle with some rosemary for some extra flavor.

Enjoy!

Nutritional information per serving: Kcal: 71, Protein: 5.5g, Carbs: 22.8g, Fats: 1.1g

16.   Orange Peach Juice

Ingredients:

1 large orange, peeled

1 large peach, pitted and halved

1 cup of watermelon, chopped

1 large Granny Smith's apple, cored

3 tbsp of fresh mint, chopped

Preparation:

Peel the orange and divide into wedges. Set aside.

Wash the peach and cut in half. Remove the pit and cut into chunks. Set aside.

Cut the watermelon lengthwise. For one cup, you will need about one large wedge. Peel and cut into chunks. Remove the seeds and set aside. Reserve the rest of the melon for some other juices.

Wash the apple and remove the core. Cut into bite-sized pieces and set aside.

Now, combine orange, peach, watermelon, and apple in a juicer and process until juiced.

Transfer to serving glasses and garnish with some fresh mint. Add some ice cubes before serving.

Enjoy!

Nutrition information per serving: Kcal: 269, Protein: 5.3g, Carbs: 78.5g, Fats: 1.3g

17.   Kiwi Lemon Juice

Ingredients:

1 whole kiwi, peeled

1 whole lemon, peeled

2 large bananas, peeled and chopped

1 cup of fresh mint, torn

1 large Red Delicious apple, cored and chopped

¼ tsp of cinnamon, ground

Preparation:

Peel the kiwi and lemon. Cut lengthwise in half and set aside.

Peel the bananas and cut into small pieces. Set aside.

Wash the mint thoroughly under cold running water. Drain and torn into small pieces. Set aside.

Wash the apple and cut lengthwise in half. Remove the core and cut into bite-sized pieces. Set aside.

Now, combine kiwi, lemon, bananas, mint, and apple in a juicer and process until well juiced. Transfer to a serving glass and stir in the cinnamon.

Add some ice and serve immediately.

Enjoy!

Nutritional information per serving: Kcal: 398, Protein: 6.1g, Carbs: 117g, Fats: 2.1g

18.   Carrot Cabbage Juice

Ingredients:

1 large carrot

1 cup of purple cabbage, chopped

2 large zucchinis, chopped

1 large red bell pepper, seeded

¼ tsp of Himalayan salt

Preparation:

Wash the carrot and cut into thick slices. Set aside.

Wash the cabbage thoroughly under cold running water and roughly chop it. Fill the measuring cup and reserve the rest for some other juice.

Peel the zucchinis and cut in half. Scrape out the seeds and cut into small chunks. Set aside.

Wash the bell pepper and cut in half. Remove the seeds and chop into small slices.

Now, combine carrot, cabbage, zucchinis, and bell pepper in a juicer and process until juiced. Add some ice cubes before serving and enjoy.

Nutritional information per serving: Kcal: 163, Protein: 11.4g, Carbs: 43.4g, Fats: 2.8g

19.   Leek Lime Juice

Ingredients:

3 large leeks, chopped

1 large lime, peeled

1 small cauliflower head, chopped

1 large zucchini, chopped

2 oz of water

Preparation:

Wash the leeks and cut into small pieces. Set aside.

Peel the lime and cut lengthwise in half. Set aside.

Trim off the outer leaves of cauliflower. Wash it and cut into small pieces. Set aside.

Peel the zucchini and cut in half. Scrape out the seeds and cut into small chunks. Set aside.

Now, combine leeks, lime, cauliflower, and zucchini in a juicer. Process until well juiced and stir in the water.

Refrigerate for 5 minutes before serving.

Nutritional information per serving: Kcal: 241, Protein: 13.2g, Carbs: 64.7g, Fats: 2.6g

20.   Avocado Peach Juice

Ingredients:

1 cup of avocado, cubed

1 large peach, chopped

1 cup of strawberries, chopped

1 large Granny Smith's apple, cored

¼ tsp of cinnamon, ground

¼ tsp of ginger, ground

2 tsp of coconut water

Preparation:

Peel the avocado and cut in half. Remove the pit and cut into small cubes. Fill the measuring cup and reserve the rest for later.

Wash the peach and cut lengthwise in half. Remove the pit and cut into bite-sized pieces. Set aside.

Wash the strawberries and remove the stems. Cut into bite-sized pieces and fill the measuring cup. Reserve the rest for later.

Wash the apple and cut in half. Remove the core and chop into small pieces. Set aside.

Now, combine avocado, peach, strawberries, and apple in a juicer and process until juiced. Transfer to a serving glass and stir in the cinnamon, ginger, and coconut water.

Refrigerate for 10 minutes before serving.

Nutritional information per serving: Kcal: 386, Protein: 6.5g, Carbs: 68.6g, Fats: 23.2g

21.   Apple Ginger Juice

Ingredients:

1 medium-sized apple, cored

1 small ginger knob, peeled

1 medium-sized carrot, sliced

1 large cucumber, sliced

1 large beet, trimmed

Preparation:

Wash the apple and remove the core. Cut into bite-sized pieces and set aside.

Peel the ginger root knob and set aside.

Wash the carrot and cucumber and cut into thick slices. Set aside.

Wash the beet and trim off the green parts. Cut into small pieces and set aside.

Now, combine carrot, apple, cucumber, beet, and ginger in a juicer and process until juiced. Transfer to serving glasses and add some ice cubes and serve immediately.

Nutrition information per serving: Kcal: 166, Protein: 4.7g, Carbs: 48.4g, Fats: 0.9g

22.   Grape Mint Juice

Ingredients:

1 cup of black grapes

1 cup of fresh mint, torn

2 cups of blueberries

1 large banana, peeled

2 tbsp of milk

¼ tsp of cinnamon, ground

Preparation:

Wash the grapes and remove the stems. Fill the measuring cup and reserve the rest in the refrigerator. Set aside.

Wash the mint thoroughly under cold running water. Drain and torn into small pieces. Set aside.

Place the blueberries in a colander. Rinse well under cold running water and drain. Set aside.

Now, combine grapes, mint, blueberries, and banana in a juicer and process until juiced. Transfer to a serving glass and stir in the milk and cinnamon.Refrigerate for 5 minutes before serving.

Nutrition information per serving: Kcal: 326, Protein: 6.2g, Carbs: 93.4g, Fats: 2.1g

23.   Arugula Pepper Juice

Ingredients:

1 cup of arugula, torn

1 large green bell pepper, seeded

1 large leek, chopped

5 large radishes, trimmed

1 large cucumber

¼ tsp of Himalayan salt

Preparation:

Wash the arugula thoroughly under cold running water and torn with hands. Set aside.

Wash the bell pepper and cut in half. Remove the seeds and chop into small pieces. Set aside.

Wash the leek and cut into small pieces. Set aside.

Wash the radishes and trim off the green parts. Cut into bite-sized pieces and set aside.

Wash the cucumber and cut into thick pieces. Set aside.

Now, process arugula, bell pepper, leek, radihes, and cucumber in a juicer. Transfer to serving glasses and stir in the salt.

Refrigerate for 5 minutes before serving.

Nutritional information per serving: Kcal: 130, Protein: 7.9g, Carbs: 37.8g, Fats: 1.1g

24. Collard Green Mint Juice

Ingredients:

1 cup of collard greens, chopped

1 cup of fresh mint, chopped

1 cup of avocado, cubed

1 large Golden Delicious apple, cored

1 oz of aloe juice

Preparation:

Peel the avocado and cut into half. Remove the pit and cut into small cubes. Fill the measuring cup and reserve the rest for later.

Combine collard greens and mint in a colander. Wash thoroughly under cold running water and slightly drain. Chop all into small pieces and set aside.

Wash the apple and cut in half. Remove the core and cut into bite-sized pieces. Set aside.

Now, combine collard greens, mint, avocado, and apple in a juicer. Process until well juiced. Transfer to a serving glass and stir in the aloe juice.

Refrigerate for 5 minutes before serving.

Nutrition information per serving: Kcal: 318, Protein: 5.6g, Carbs: 47.7g, Fats: 22.7g

25.   Apple Asparagus Juice

Ingredients:

1 large Red Delicious apple, cored

1 cup of wild asparagus, trimmed

1 cup of fresh spinach, torn

1 cup of collard greens, torn

1 cup of mustard greens, torn

2 oz of water

Preparation:

Wash the apple and cut in half. Remove the core and cut into bite-sized pieces. Set aside.

Combine spinach, collard greens, and mustard greens in a large colander. Wash under cold running water and drain. Torn with hands and set aside.

Now, combine apple spinach, collard greens, and mustard greens in a juicer and process until well juiced. Transfer to serving glasses and stir in the water. Refrigerate for 10 minutes before serving.

Nutritional information per serving: Kcal: 207, Protein: 16.1g, Carbs: 58.6g, Fats: 2.5g

26.   Orange Apple Juice

Ingredients:

1 large orange, peeled

1 small green apple, cored

1 cup of strawberries, halved

3 oz of coconut water

¼ tsp of vanilla extract

Preparation:

Peel the orange and divide into wedges. Set aside.

Wash the apple and remove the core. Cut into bite-sized pieces and set aside.

Place the strawberries in a colander and wash under cold running water. Drain and cut in half. Set aside.

Now, combine orange, apple, and strawberries in a juicer and process until juiced.

Transfer to serving glasses and add some ice before serving.

Nutritional information per serving: Kcal: 211, Protein: 3.5g, Carbs: 58g, Fats: 0.9g

27.   Lime Kale Juice

Ingredients:

1 large lime, peeled

1 cup of kale, torn

1 large artichoke head

1 large cucumber

A handful of spinach, torn

Preparation:

Peel the lime and cut lengthwise in half. Set aside.

Wash the kale and spinach thoroughly under cold running water. Drain and torn with hands. Set aside.

Trim off the outer leaves of the artichoke using a sharp knife. Cut into small pieces and set aside.

Wash the cucumber and cut into thick slices. Set aside.

Now, combine, lime, kale, artichoke, cucumber, and spinach in a juicer and process until juiced.

Transfer to serving glasses and add some ice before serving.

Nutritional information per serving: Kcal: 117, Protein: 11.1g, Carbs: 38.6g, Fats: 1.3g

28.   Cantaloupe Apple Juice

Ingredients:

1 cup of cantaloupe, seeded

1 large green apple, cored

1 cup of watermelon, seeded

1 medium-sized banana

¼ tsp of vanilla extract

2 oz of water

Preparation:

Cut the cantaloupe in half. Scoop out the seeds and flesh. Cut two wedges and peel them. Chop into chunks and set aside. Reserve the rest of the cantaloupe in a refrigerator.

Wash the apple and remove the core. Cut into bite-sized pieces and set aside.

Cut the watermelon lengthwise. For one cup, you will need about one large wedge. Peel and cut into chunks. Remove the seeds and set aside. Reserve the rest of the melon for some other juices.

Peel the banana and chop into small chunks. Set aside.

Now, combine cantaloupe, apple, watermelon, and banana in a juicer and process until juiced.

Transfer to serving glasses and stir in the vanilla extract and water. Add some ice and serve immediately.

Enjoy!

Nutritional information per serving: Kcal: 294, Protein: 4.6g, Carbs: 83.3g, Fats: 1.3g

29.   Cucumber Lemon Juice

Ingredients:

1 large cucumber, sliced

1 large lemon, peeled

2 cups of fresh cherries, pitted

1 medium-sized Granny smith apple, cored

2 oz of water

Preparation:

Wash the cucumber and cut into thick slices. Set aside.

Peel the lemon and cut lengthwise in half. Set aside.

Using a colander, wash the cherries under cold running water. Cut in half and remove the pits. Set aside.

Wash the apple and remove the core. Cut into bite-sized pieces and set aside.

Now, combine cucumber, lemon, cherry, and apple in a juicer and process until juiced. Transfer to serving glasses and stir in the water. Add few ice cubes before serving.

Nutritional information per serving: Kcal: 296, Protein: 6.6g, Carbs: 88.4g, Fats: 1.4g

30.   Asparagus Banana Juice

Ingredients:

1 cup of asparagus, trimmed and chopped

1 large banana, peeled and chunked

1 cup of celery, chopped

1 small ginger knob, 1-inch thick

1 oz of water

Preparation:

Wash the asparagus and trim off the woody ends. Cut into bite-sized pieces and set aside.

Peel the banana and cut into small chunks. Set aside.

Wash the celery stalks and cut into bite-sized pieces. Fill the measuring cup and reserve the rest for some other juice.

Peel the ginger knob and chop it.

Now, combine asparagus, banana, celery, and ginger in a juicer and process until juiced. Transfer to a serving glass and stir in the water.

Add some crushed ice and serve immediately.

Nutrition information per serving: Kcal: 138, Protein: 5.3g, Carbs: 40.3g, Fats: 0.8g

31.   Cranberry Blackberry Juice

Ingredients:

1 cup of cranberries

1 cup of blackberries

1 cup of cantaloupe, diced

1 small Golden Delicious apple, cored

¼ tsp of cinnamon, ground

¼ tsp of ginger, ground

Preparation:

Combine cranberries and blackberries in a large colander. Rinse well under cold running water and drain. Set aside.

Cut the cantaloupe in half. Scrape out the seeds and cut one large wedge. Peel and dice into small pieces. Fill the measuring cup and wrap the rest in a plastic foil. Refrigerate for later.

Wash the apple cut lengthwise in half. Remove the core and cut into bite-sized pieces. Set aside.

Now, combine cranberries, blackberries, cantaloupe, and apple in a juicer and process until well juiced. Transfer to a serving glass and stir in the cinnamon and ginger.

Add some crushed ice and serve immediately.

Enjoy!

Nutrition information per serving: Kcal: 169, Protein: 4.1g, Carbs: 56.3g, Fats: 1.3g

32.   Fennel Spinach Juice

Ingredients:

1 cup of fennel, trimmed and chopped

1 cup of spinach, torn

2 large red bell peppers, seeds removed

1cup of cucumber, sliced

¼ tsp of salt

¼ tsp of cayenne pepper, ground

Preparation:

Trim off the fennel stalks and outer wilted layers. Wash and chop the fennel into bite-sized pieces. Fill the measuring cup and reserve the rest for later. Set aside.

Rinse the spinach thoroughly under cold running water. Drain and torn into small pieces. Fill the measuring cup and reserve the rest in the refrigerator.

Wash the bell peppers and cut each lengthwise in half. Remove the stem and seeds. Chop into small pieces and set aside.

Wash the cucumber and cut into thin slices. Fill the measuring cup and reserve the rest for later.

Now, combine fennel, spinach, bell peppers, and cucumber in a juicer and process until juiced. Transfer to a serving glass and stir in the salt and cayenne pepper.

Serve cold.

Nutrition information per serving: Kcal: 125, Protein: 10.6g, Carbs: 35.65g, Fats: 2.1g

33.   Pepper Orange Juice

Ingredients:

1 cup of pumpkin, cubed

1 large yellow bell pepper, seeded

1 large orange, peeled

1 large lime, peeled

1 small rosemary sprig

Preparation:

Wash the bell pepper and cut in half. Remove the seeds and cut into small slices. Set aside.

Peel the orange and divide into wedges. Set aside.

Peel the pumpkin and cut in half. Scoop out the seeds using a spoon. Cut one large wedge and peel it. Cut into small chunks and fill the measuring cup. Reserve the rest for some other juice.

Peel the lime and cut lengthwise in half. Set aside.

Now, combine bell pepper, orange, pumpkin, and lime in a juicer and process until juiced. Transfer to serving glasses and sprinkle with some rosemary to taste.

Refrigerate for 10 minutes before serving.

Nutrition information per serving: Kcal: 149, Protein: 4.9g, Carbs: 44.6g, Fats: 0.7g

34.   Peach Apple Juice

Ingredients:

1 cup of watermelon, cubed

2 large peaches, pitted

1 large green apple, cored

5 fresh cherries, pitted

3 oz of coconut water

Preparation:

Wash the peaches and cut in half. Remove the pits and cut into bite-sized pieces. Set aside.

Wash the apple and cut in half. Remove the core and cut into bite-sized pieces. Set aside.

Cut the watermelon lengthwise. For one cup, you will need about one large wedge. Peel and cut into chunks. Remove the seeds and set aside. Reserve the rest of the melon for some other juices.

Wash the cherries and cut in half. Remove the pits and set aside.

Now, process peaches, apple, watermelon, and cherries in a juicer. Transfer to serving glasses and stir in the coconut water. Add some ice and serve immediately.

Nutritional information per serving: Kcal: 276, Protein: 5.4g, Carbs: 47.6g, Fats: 1.6g

35.　Apricot Swiss Chard Juice

Ingredients:

3 whole apricots, pitted

1 cup of Swiss chard, torn

1 whole grapefruit, peeled and wedged

1 medium-sized apple, cored

1 tbsp of liquid honey

¼ tsp of ginger, ground

Preparation:

Wash the apricots and cut into halves. Chop all into small pieces and set aside.

Rinse the Swiss chard thoroughly under cold running water. Drain and torn into small pieces. Set aside.

Peel the grapefruit and divide into wedges. Cut each wedge in half and set aside.

Wash the apple and cut lengthwise in half. Remove the core and chop into bite-sized pieces. Set aside.

Now, combine apricots, Swiss chard, grapefruit, and apple in a juicer and process until juiced. Transfer to a serving glass and stir in the honey and ginger.

Add few ice cubes and serve immediately.

Nutrition information per serving: Kcal: 212, Protein: 4.7g, Carbs: 61.9g, Fats: 1.1g

36.   Brussels Sprout Carrot Juice

Ingredients:

1 cup of Brussels sprouts, trimmed

1 large carrot, sliced

1 large artichoke, peeled and chopped

1 cup of fresh celery, chopped

1 cup of turnip greens, chopped

1 large green apple, cored

½ tsp of turmeric, ground

2 oz of water

Preparation:

Trim off the outer leaves of the Brussels sprouts and wash them thoroughly. Cut in half and set aside.

Wash the carrot and cut into thin slices. Set aside.

Using a sharp knife, trim off the outer leaves of the artichoke. Cut into small pieces and set aside.

Wash the celery and chop it into bite-sized pieces. Set aside.

Wash the apple and cut in half. Remove the core and cut into bite-sized pieces. Set aside.

Wash the turnip greens thoroughly and torn with hands. Set aside.

Now, combine Brussels sprouts, carrot, artichoke, celery, turnip greens, and apple in a juicer. Process until well juiced and transfer to serving glasses. Stir in the turmeric and water. Add some ice before serving.

Nutritional information per serving: Kcal: 205, Protein: 11.3g, Carbs: 66.7g, Fats: 1.4g

37.　Zucchini Celery Juice

Ingredients:

1 medium-sized zucchini, sliced

1 cup of celery, chopped

1 cup of purple cabbage, torn

1 cup of cucumber, sliced

¼ tsp of turmeric, ground

¼ tsp of salt

Preparation:

Wash the zucchini and cut into thin slices. Set aside.

Wash the celery and chop into bite-sized pieces. Set aside.

Rinse the purple cabbage under cold running water. Drain and torn into small pieces and set aside.

Wash the cucumber and cut into slices. Fill the measuring cup and reserve the rest for later.

Now, combine cabbage, zucchini, celery, and cucumber in a juicer and process until juiced. Transfer to a serving glass and stir in the turmeric and salt.

Refrigerate for 5 minutes before serving.

Enjoy!

Nutrition information per serving: Kcal: 62, Protein: 4.7g, Carbs: 17.5g, Fats: 1g

38.   Raspberry Lemon Juice

Ingredients:

1 cup of raspberries

1 large lemon, peeled

1 cup of apricots, pitted and chopped

1 cup of cucumber, chopped

1 medium-sized orange, peeled

2 oz of water

Preparation:

Place the raspberries in a colander and wash thoroughly under cold running water. Drain and set aside.

Peel the lemon and cut lengthwise in half. Set aside.

Wash the apricots and cut in half. Remove the pits and cut into bite-sized pieces. Fill the measuring cup and reserve the rest for some other juice.

Peel the orange and divide into wedges. Set aside.

Now, combine, raspberries, lemon, apricots, and orange in a juicer and process until juiced.

Transfer to serving glasses and stir in the water. Add some ice and serve immediately.

Nutritional information per serving: Kcal: 166, Protein: 6g, Carbs: 55.7g, Fats: 1.8g

39.   Watercress Lemon Juice

Ingredients:

1 cup of watercress

2 large leeks

1 large lemon, peeled

1 cup of watermelon, seeded

1 cup of beet greens

2 oz of water

Preparation:

Wash the watercress and beet greens thoroughly under cold running water and torn with hands. Set aside.

Wash the leeks and cut into 1-inch pieces. Set aside.

Peel the lemon and cut lengthwise in half. Set aside.

Cut the watermelon lengthwise. For two cups, you will need about two large wedges. Peel and cut into chunks. Remove the seeds and set aside. Reserve the rest of the melon for some other juices.

Now, combine watercress, leeks, lemon, watermelon, and beet greens in a juicer and process until juiced.

Transfer to serving glasses and stir in the water. Add some ice cubes and serve immediately.

Nutrition information per serving: Kcal: 156, Protein: 5.9g, Carbs: 44.2g, Fats: 1.1g

40.   Ginger Carrot Juice

Ingredients:

1 small ginger knob, peeled and chopped

1 medium-sized carrot, sliced

1 cup of watermelon, diced

1 medium-sized wedge of honeydew melon

1 small banana, chunked

Preparation:

Peel the ginger and cut into small pieces. Set aside.

Wash and peel the carrot. Cut into thin slices and set aside.

Cut the top of the watermelon. Cut lengthwise in half and then cut one large wedge. Peel it and cut into small cubes. Remove the seeds and fill the measuring cup. Wrap the rest in a plastic foil and refrigerate for later.

Cut the melon in half. Cut one large wedge and peel the peel it. Cut into small pieces and set aside. Wrap the rest of the melon in a plastic foil and refrigerate for some other juice.

Peel the banana and cut into chunks. Set aside.

Now, combine, ginger, carrot, watermelon, honeydew melon, and banana in a juicer. Process until juiced.

Transfer to a serving glass and add some crushed ice before serving.

Enjoy!

Nutrition information per serving: Kcal: 188, Protein: 3.4g, Carbs: 52.8g, Fats: 0.9g

41.   Apple Banana Juice

Ingredients:

1 large Granny Smith's apple, cored and chopped

1 large banana, peeled

1 cup of strawberries, chopped

1 cup of fresh mint, torn

2 oz of water

Preparation:

Wash the apple and cut lengthwise in half. Remove the core and chop into small pieces. Set aside.

Peel the banana and cut into small chunks. Set aside.

Wash the strawberries and remove the stems. Cut into bite-sized pieces and fill the measuring cup. Reserve the rest in the refrigerator. Set aside.

Wash the mint thoroughly under cold running water. Drain and torn into small pieces. Set aside.

Now, combine apple, banana, strawberries, and mint in a juicer. Process until well juiced. Transfer to a serving glass and stir in the water.

Add some ice and serve immediately.

Nutrition information per serving: Kcal: 245, Protein: 4.3g, Carbs: 73.8g, Fats: 1.5g

42.   Brussels Sprout Broccoli Juice

Ingredients:

1 cup of Brussels sprouts, trimmed

1 cup of fresh broccoli

1 large wedge of honeydew melon

1 cup of parsnip, trimmed

1 medium-sized apple, cored

2 oz of water

Preparation:

Wash the Brussels sprouts and trim off the outer leaves. Cut in half and set aside.

Wash the broccoli and chop into small pieces. Set aside.

Cut the honeydew melon lengthwise in half. Scoop out the seeds using a spoon. Cut one large wedge and peel it. Cut into small chunks and place in a bowl. Wrap the rest of the melon in a plastic foil and refrigerate.

Wash the parsnips and cut into thick slices. Fill into the measuring cup and reserve the rest for some other juice. Set aside.

Wash the apple and remove the core. Cut into bite-sized pieces and set aside.

Now, process Brussels sprouts, broccoli, honeydew melon, parsnips, and apple in a juicer.

Transfer to serving glasses and stir in the water. Add some ice and serve!

Nutrition information per serving: Kcal: 251, Protein: 8.7g, Carbs: 75.1g, Fats: 1.5g

43.   Pumpkin Apple Juice

Ingredients:

1 cup of pumpkin

1 medium-sized yellow apple, cored

1 large zucchini chunks

1 large lemon, peeled

1 medium-sized banana

2 oz of water

Preparation:

Peel the pumpkin and cut in half. Scoop out the seeds using a spoon. Cut one large wedge and peel it. Cut into small chunks and set aside. Reserve the rest for later.

Wash the apple and remove the core. Cut into bite-sized pieces and set aside.

Peel the zucchini and cut in half. Scrape out the seeds with a spoon. Cut into chunks and set aside.

Peel the lemon and cut lengthwise in half. Set aside.

Peel the banana and cut into small chunks. Set aside.

Now, process pumpkin, apple, zucchini, lemon, and banana in a juicer. Transfer to serving glasses and stir in the water.

Add some ice and serve immediately.

Nutrition information per serving: Kcal: 254, Protein: 7.5g, Carbs: 72.9g, Fats: 1.9g

44.   Parsley Artichoke Juice

Ingredients:

1 cup of fresh parsley, torn

1 medium-sized artichoke, chopped

2 medium-sized Roma tomatoes, chopped

1 cup of Romaine lettuce, torn

¼ tsp of salt

¼ tsp of dried oregano, ground

Preparation:

Combine parsley and lettuce in a large colander. Rinse well under cold running water and drain. Torn into small pieces and set aside.

Wash the artichoke trim off the outer leaves. Chop into bite-sized pieces and fill the measuring cup. Reserve the rest in the refrigerator. Set aside.

Wash the tomatoes and place in a bowl. Chop into small pieces and make sure to reserve the tomato juice while cutting. Set aside.

Now, combine parsley, artichoke, tomatoes, and lettuce in a juicer and process until juiced. Transfer to a serving glass and stir in the salt and oregano.

Refrigerate for 5 minutes before serving.

Enjoy!

Nutrition information per serving: Kcal: 82, Protein: 8.7g, Carbs: 28.3g, Fats: 1.3g

45.   Spinach Lime Juice

Ingredients:

1 cup of fresh spinach, torn

1 large lime, peeled

1 cup of avocado, pitted and chopped

1 large cucumber, sliced

1 large lemon, peeled

1 small ginger knob, peeled

3 oz of water

Preparation:

Wash the spinach thoroughly and torn with hands. Set aside.

Peel the lemon and lime. Cut lengthwise in half and set aside.

Peel the avocado and cut in half. Remove the pit and chop into chunks. Set aside.

Wash the cucumber and cut into thick slices. Set aside.

Peel the ginger knob and set aside.

Now, combine lime, spinach, avocado, cucumber, lemon, and ginger in a juicer. Process until juiced and transfer to serving glasses. Stir in the water and refrigerate for 5 minutes before serving.

Enjoy!

Nutritional information per serving: Kcal: 269, Protein: 6.7g, Carbs: 35g, Fats: 22.6g

ADDITIONAL TITLES FROM THIS AUTHOR

70 Effective Meal Recipes to Prevent and Solve Being Overweight: Burn Fat Fast by Using Proper Dieting and Smart Nutrition

By

Joe Correa CSN

48 Acne Solving Meal Recipes: The Fast and Natural Path to Fixing Your Acne Problems in Less Than 10 Days!

By

Joe Correa CSN

41 Alzheimer's Preventing Meal Recipes: Reduce or Eliminate Your Alzheimer's Condition in 30 Days or Less!

By

Joe Correa CSN

70 Effective Breast Cancer Meal Recipes: Prevent and Fight Breast Cancer with Smart Nutrition and Powerful Foods

By

Joe Correa CSN

www.ingramcontent.com/pod-product-compliance
Lightning Source LLC
Chambersburg PA
CBHW030245030426
42336CB00009B/268